Run

at

Any Age

A Beginner's Guide for Adults

Carol M Green

Run
At
Any Age

A Beginner's Guide
for Adults

ISBN: 978-1546641209

DEDICATION

This book is dedicated to my running peers, many of
whom began running as adults and not-so-young adults,
and to my running proteges.
May you ever find joy in the run.

Contents

Section III - Trouble Shooting   **87**

Section IV - Runners' Speech   **115**

ACKNOWLEDGMENTS

Special thanks to Judith Ann Kidd, Renda Ware, Peggy Thomson, Melanie Millner, and Maria Weber.

To Judith, my editor, for her sharp eye and frank feedback as she ever encourages me to follow my dreams.

To Renda, Peggy, and Mel, for their invaluable input and willingness to try.

To Maria, my teammate, for her runner's perspective and warrior's heart.

Introduction

The purpose of this book is not to convince you, the reader, that you should begin running. You have already come to that realization. You may, however, have some doubts about your ability to become a runner.

The purpose of this book is 1) to encourage and convince you that you CAN begin running given you have a clear bill of health from your doctor, 2) to give you information that will help you get started, 3) to provide tips and techniques to help you endure when the physical or mental going gets tough, and 4) to help you obtain benefits and satisfaction that only a runner will understand.

This book is for anyone who is anxious about running, but especially for women who have neglected their physical well-being while providing for the day-to-day needs of those they love. You know who you are and you want to be healthier – not so much for yourself, but for those you love. You want to live a long and active life so you will be here to care for, celebrate with, and cheer on your loved ones, young and old.

You know you should, but you aren't convinced you can. Let's begin by dispelling some of the myths you have heard or created about running. Let's begin slowly and wisely. Let's begin with the right tools to be successful. Let's begin with the support and encouragement of other runners.

Let's begin!

Section I

First Things First

This section is intended to help you get started. What do you need to know before you begin? What physical and mental preparations are necessary before heading out on your first run? How will you stay on this new path you have determined to follow?

As always, if you are just beginning to exercise, check with your physician to be certain you are ready to become a runner. It is very likely you will get the green light to begin.

Carol M Green

It's Okay to Run

So, you think you want to be a runner? Perhaps you are not sure. Perhaps you don't know if you should be a runner. What if you are slow? What if you have poor running form? What if others, friends and strangers, think you are silly for trying? What if you have to take a walking break and somebody sees you?

Well, all runners know this little secret. You are going to have to get over yourself! Before you get offended, please read on ...

I was once a non-runner. I became a runner at the tender age of 47. Runners run. That's all there is to it. Non-runners who wish they were runners tend to come up with all kinds of excuses why they can't, shouldn't, or won't run. I know. Before I began running I used every excuse not to run.

"I'm too old to start." Yep, I said that.

"I don't like to run." I said that one a lot!

"It hurts to run." Yes, it does.

And then there is this one ...

"I don't want anybody to see me trying to run."

Well, for those of you who are hanging onto this excuse, I have some news for you. NOBODY is looking at a runner and thinking this ...

"Boy, that runner sure does look stupid."

Nor this ...

"That runner shouldn't be running. She's too big, old, fat, short, weak ..." Insert your own negative adjective if you like. Nobody is thinking any of those things.

In fact, those non-runners driving by in their cars with their car snacks by their side are most surely thinking something like this:

"I wish I were a runner. I wish I was strong enough, brave enough, in shape enough ... to run."

I know. I was once one of those non-runners. They are having thoughts more like this ...

"Wow, I really should stop eating chips. I wonder how long she has been running? How far can she run? I should really get more exercise. Maybe someday I'll run, too."

The runners who happen to be in a car or stuck at their desk job while you are running are thinking ...

"Look! There is a runner! Maybe we could be running buddies!"

"I'm jealous. I wish I was running right now."

"Wow. I hope I can still run when I'm as old as that guy!"

"I am so proud of that runner out there getting in shape and taking care of her heart and lungs! Way to go, Runner!"

The hesitation to be caught running is natural. When I began running my running buddy and I would search for the most hidden routes we could find to avoid being seen. We didn't want anyone to criticize our form or see how miserable we looked with red faces and sweat glistening all over, but I got over that. I have learned that if I admire other runners when I am not running, then surely others are not judging me while I am on the run.

It doesn't matter if you have great running form or a cute outfit. The car riders cannot tell how fast or slow you are moving and they don't care. They only know that you are out there putting one foot in front of the other. They respect your efforts, especially if they are also a runner.

Try this:

Repeat in your mind the following words, "I am a runner. I am improving my health. I am strong. I can run." Crush the negative thoughts and hesitancy by replacing them with positive affirmations and then get over yourself and just run!

Carol M Green

Get Over Your Fear

Beginning running can be scary, I will admit. There are so many unknowns. You might wonder if running is something you should even attempt. What if it hurts? What if I'm not very good at it? What if I don't love it? Having questions is no reason to avoid trying. My mother used to tell me, "You'll never know unless you try." Well, I tried and now I know.

What if it hurts?

I guarantee it is going to hurt. There are a lot of things in life that hurt, many of them should be avoided. However, there are many things that cause us pain that actually improve our lives. Running is one of those things. I expound upon this subject in depth in my book about different kinds of pain and our relationship with that pain, The Hard Run: Painful Lessons from a Running Granny. I tell all new runners, "It's okay to hurt."

What if you aren't very good at it?

You very likely will not be good at running – at least not at first. That's okay. You weren't good at walking or crawling when you first tried those things, but you didn't

21

quit and look how well you can walk now. Give it some time. You may never be a fast runner, but you can be a stronger runner and stronger person if you stick with it.

What if you don't love it?

You may never love running. Even if that love does happen running often takes a little time to grow on you. While you are waiting for that fondness to develop you might as well keep running, because it is good for you. I often say, "I don't love running. Running loves me!" It improves my life in many ways.

I am certain there are more questions that soon to be runners may be pondering. What happens if I get injured? We will address injuries, treatment, and prevention in later chapters. What if I ruin my knees? You won't. What if …

Anticipating what could go wrong is often more terrible than the actual activity. So, give it a go. "You'll never know unless you try."

Try this:

Acknowledge that you are going to have some apprehensions. Ask yourself, "Will I survive?" If the answer is yes, then be courageous and get moving!

What Will You Wear?

Congratulations! You've made the mental commitment to begin running and you have worked to conquer your fear. You are still reading this book, and that's a good sign. It's almost time to get started. Now what? It is time to don some gear and hit the road.

What will you wear on your …

Feet - It's all about the shoes. They are the most important piece of equipment for any runner. You will find that runners spend more time talking about their shoes than their running playlists, favorite smoothie recipes, or even the weather. You can begin without a fancy new pair of runners, but if you plan to continue running it would be wise to visit a running store and get a good fit. Why do you need a running store? Running stores are typically owned and operated by – you guessed it – runners! They are interested in supporting you as a runner and understand the value of the right fit. They have the expertise to help you find the best shoe for you. It's never about making a sale today. If you are successful, the shoe sales will naturally follow.

Good shoes may cost a little more than clearance gym shoes at an all-purpose shoe store, but they will be worth it and your feet, legs, hips, and knees will thank you!

Socks will take some experimenting. Some runners don't wear socks. Other runners like a thick sock, while some are interested in the appearance. Don't spend a lot of money on new socks right away. I buy mine in the "six pair for $8 packs" and I like them. It's just a matter of preference. Unless it's below 20 degrees, your toes will be fine. Blisters are a bigger concern than cold toes, so make sure you wear socks that fit. Shoes should be tight enough to prevent slipping and rubbing. Your toes will warm up in a couple miles. Blisters will plague you much longer than that!

The rest of your attire is up to you. There is no need to purchase a new wardrobe before beginning. Runners can wear anything that keeps them comfortable.

Here are a few ideas ...

Legs - I prefer spandex (American term for elastane) on my legs in hot or cold weather because it keeps me covered and prevents chafing! Yes, we runners talk about things like that. However, a pair of sweatpants or gym shorts will do. Don't use a lack of spandex as an excuse to delay your new running adventure. Pockets come in handy for carrying car keys, phones, and Chapstick. I have found that my legs can weather the cold or hot better than the rest of me, so I don't need to change up my running pants along with the seasons. On chilly days, a second layer of running tights or sweatpants may be needed. Do what feels best, but remember, you won't be shedding the second layer unless you want to take time to remove and retie your shoes.

Torso - Winter running can be deceiving. Layer up and be prepared to shed some clothing once you have been on the move for a little while. Wear a long sleeve wicking shirt next to your body and another layer over that. The first few minutes may be frigid, but it's called a "warm up" for a reason. Once you get your heart pumping the cold won't be so bothersome. A hoodie sweatshirt is great for temps in the mid and lower 30's. It can be removed and tied around your waist if you get too warm. A second, long sleeve or short sleeve shirt is sufficient when temps climb into the 40's.

In warmer seasons, a light T-shirt or athletic wear made of wicking fabric will be sufficient. Again, don't wait for the perfect outfit before you begin.

Ladies, you're going to want a sports bra. Trust me.

Head - I prefer a headband over a cap for this one reason. When I get warm, I can remove the headband, twist it in two and wear it on my wrist. It doesn't get lost and I don't worry if it was tucked safely in a pocket. The hood of a sweatshirt can be pulled over the headband if the weather gets very nasty.

Eyes - Sunglasses, always. They will protect your eyes from sun, snow, sleet and the occasional obnoxious flying bug! Add a running cap to help you hide from passersby if you have not yet conquered self-consciousness.

Hands - Wear a pair of gloves that are easy to discard or store in a pocket. Cheap knitted gloves are my favorite. You can cut a thumb out for cell phone texts and photo opportunities. They can be stowed in a pocket or easily carried along your route. Better yet, map your route with a loop about two miles into the run. You'll be ready to shed a few items and you can come back and pick them up while cooling down on your way home. I know one runner that wears socks on his hands during cold weather rather than gloves because he likes to keep his fingers snuggled up together.

Phone – I know it's not a body part, but phones have become a part of us. You will find it especially helpful for timing your workout, tracking your route, monitoring your pace, photo journaling your run, and taking pictures of dogs at large whose owners are breaking leash laws! I prefer a small running belt or pocket to an armband because I can't read my phone when it's strapped to my arm. Experiment to find what works best for you.

Try this:

Begin with what you have and let experience teach you what you prefer. When the temperatures drop, experiment with your running gear by mapping a short route that loops back to your home. You can warm up with more layers and then shed them when you run back by. Do this until you have discovered the best cold weather running outfit for you.

Remember, the best running outfit is the one that you wear while you run. It helps if it looks good, but cold weather running calls for flexibility and adaptation. You can save the hot pink tees and flashy running socks for summer sunshine.

Carol M Green

Your First Run

Let's assume you have already been exercising or that you have at least visited with your doctor and received the okay to take up running as a form of exercise. (If not, go ahead and make that visit. He will probably tell you it's a good idea and wish you the best.) You are cleared to run, you have a decent pair of shoes and something to cover the rest of your body. It's time to run!

Find a route that is smooth and measurable. A high school track is ideal because it was built for running. Walking paths offer a great surface on which to run, but they may be busy with foot traffic and onlookers. That's okay because you have read the previous chapters and know that onlookers are more likely to admire than criticize. Walking paths are going to be more difficult to measure, but a watch or phone with GPS capabilities will help. Country roads are often laid out in half and one mile grids with power poles that offer shorter measurements for your first run. Be certain to run on the left side of the road facing oncoming traffic for safety purposes. Like I tell my cross country runners, "You want to be able to see the person that is going to run over you!"

Begin with a brisk warm up walk for ¼ to ½ mile or about 5 minutes. Swing your arms, get your heart rate going, and tell yourself, "Today, I will be a runner."

Stretch! (See the next section of this book.)

Choose a distance. This may be from one power pole to the next or one lap around the track. Determine to run that distance before taking a walk break. Go as slowly as necessary to finish the goal but quickly enough that you are out of breath and uncomfortable when you have reached the goal. Take a short walk break, never farther than the distance you just ran, and then repeat.

Your first run might not be spectacular. Don't be discouraged. You will quickly improve.

Try this:

Set a timer for 30 – 40 minutes on your watch or phone. Do the run/walk exercise for the full 30 – 40 minutes. Then take some time to walk it out and stretch. (Important! Read the next section on stretching before you begin.)

Learn to Stretch

One reason I run is that I am impatient. Running is the quickest way I can think of to get in a good workout. I have learned, however, that if I want to keep running I have to take time to stretch. I've got a little sciatic nerve (Okay, sciatic nerves are very large!) that bothers me when I forget to stretch. If neglected too long, it becomes more than bothersome and I have to seek the help of a massage therapist to find relief.

 Among the benefits of stretching are:

Injury prevention – While a pinched sciatic nerve is painful, I would not consider it an injury. It's a condition that needs attention. Injuries that occur due to lack of stretching are more likely to be muscle cramping and tears. A calf or hamstring tear will stop you short and necessitate rest and time for healing. A few minutes of stretching after warming up and again after a cool down will help to keep you on your feet.

Loosens tight muscles – When you begin running, you are likely to find that your calf, quadriceps, hamstring, and even lower back muscles are letting you know they are overworked and underpaid. Listen to them. They are warning you of impending injury – and they hurt.

31

Sufficient stretching of these muscle groups will help to ease the discomfort and avoid injuries that can sideline you.

Increased flexibility and balance – Stretching and yoga poses can improve not only your flexibility, but your balance may benefit, too. Better balance is a benefit of running as it strengthens muscles. Proper stretching adds to that balance benefit.

Relaxation – I have learned that stretching before bedtime helps me relax and get a better night's sleep. Even if you have taken time to stretch after your workout, a few minutes before bed will help work out the kinks in fatigued muscles and allow them to regenerate while you sleep.

Time to reflect – A few minutes of stretching or yoga allows the mind to settle and reflect on the day or run. While holding a stretch, ask yourself, "What went well this time? What didn't go so well? How could I make my day, run, or experience better?" You may discover that stretching can be a valuable activity after any pursuit that requires physical or mental effort.

Try this:

Learn effective stretching for the following muscle groups – calves, quads, hamstrings, glutes, back, and shoulders by researching online videos or enrolling in a yoga class. Spend a few minutes after your warmup, after your run, and before bedtime getting all those tired muscle groups stretched out.

Take a Breath

Breathing. We all must to do it, and fortunately, it's an involuntary action so it doesn't usually take much thought. Keep that in mind and don't overthink your breathing on the run. Unfortunately, as breathing becomes difficult or labored as it often does with exercise, it is easy to overthink or panic. Don't. Staying relaxed will go a long way in helping you get the precious oxygen your brain and muscles require.

There are a few indications that you need to relax or change the way you are breathing. Let's consider some of them.

You have a side stitch or pain in one side of your waist or lower ribs. You may be breathing too rapidly. Relax your shoulders and inhale a big breath through your nose or mouth. Then release it slowly, counting 1, 2, 3, 4. Repeat. Practice this technique for some distance until the discomfort in your side subsides. When possible, slow your inhale to two to four counts, as well.

Your lungs feel as if they can't expand enough to accommodate all the air they need. You are most likely not breathing deeply enough. Your ribs can only expand so far. You need to use your diaphragm to expand your chest cavity downward. Place one hand on your stomach and feel it expand outward as you inhale deeply. It may seem counterproductive – making your stomach bigger – but you'll run longer and your resting stomach may even get smaller.

You sound as if you are breathing too hard and it makes you nervous that you are working too hard. Don't panic. Turn on your running music and drown out those heavy breaths. When you can't hear your breathing, you can better evaluate how you feel. You will likely discover that you are not breathing nearly so hard as it sounds.

You've tried all these tricks and it still feels as if you can't get enough air. Slow down. You may be running too fast for your fitness level. Take a walk break if necessary. Remember, the goal is to keep running. If a slower pace keeps you moving then go ahead and take it slow.

Try this:

On each run, take a few moments to evaluate your breathing. Are you experiencing any of the following?

> You have a side stitch.
> Your lungs feel as if they can't expand enough.
> You are breathing rapidly in and out.
> The sound of your breathing is alarming.

You may have a tendency towards one or more of these breathing mistakes. When the going gets tough, implement one of the above techniques and make a mental note of how it works for you. When you feel like you can't go farther, check your breathing, control it, and keep going.

Make it Fun

Running, or any other form of cardio exercise, is not easy. There will be discomfort, and sweat, and tired and sore muscles. You will want to quit. If you are going to stick with a new training plan you better find a way to enjoy it. It's much easier to spend time doing things you love than things you detest, but what if you don't love running? I don't love running. Running loves me! Surprised? I run for the benefits. On occasion, I truly enjoy running, but I can't say I love it. That's why I find things to enjoy on the run.

Music – Download some of your favorite songs for your next lonely run. You can belt out the lyrics while you trot along. You'll be surprised how good you sound as a backup singer to your favorite band.

Photo Shoot – I always carry my phone for safety reasons. I have never had to call for help, but I have snapped a shot of a sunset or waterfowl I spied along the way. Take a picture of that big hill you just conquered and share it with the world.

Document – Make a list of all the strange and exciting things you find along your route. Why is there an empty toothpaste tube in the barrow pit by a corn field? How long has that squished frog, snake, or mouse been there? Are those cows staring at you? What are they thinking? Recording interesting things that you observed during your run will help you look forward to your next running adventure.

Achieve – If you are a competitive sort, set some time, pace, or mileage goals and check them off your list as you conquer each challenge. You'll find great satisfaction as you complete each new goal. Keep a running journal and add up your miles over a week, a month, or even a year.

Look good – One of my mottos is, "Looking good is half the battle." Find something fun to wear on the run that you wouldn't wear anywhere else like crazy socks or neon tights. Share a picture of your outfit of the day on social media. You'll be surprised how many new running friends you will gain.

Walk – Give yourself permission to walk. If you need a break, take one. Don't make it a long break. When you have caught your breath, you can run farther.

Obstacle course – Once a running buddy and I ran on a dirt road through some fields. When we turned a corner, we found that there were sprinkle pipes across our path. We thought about turning around, but decided to jump over them. We laughed and jumped for a half mile! Find something unusual to run around, jump or crawl over, or even wade through.

Write about it – You are bound to have an experience worth sharing. Go ahead, tell the world about it on social media, a blog, in your running journal, in your personal journal for posterity, or get truly ambitious and write a book!

Try this:

Set a goal to implement one of the above "fun tricks" on your next run, then make a mental or written note comparing it to previous workouts. What was effective? How did it help you enjoy or stay focused on your run? Will you use this same trick in the future? Perhaps it didn't work as well as you anticipated. What could make it work better?

Get a Buddy

Running buddies are motivators who can save you from yourself and make your run more fun. Whether you are just starting out or you have been running for a while and need a little motivation, a running buddy can help you stick to your training plan – even if that plan is simply to keep moving. Here are a few examples of ways the buddy system works for me.

Training Buddy – You and this buddy have committed to a race. You are following a training plan with regular and specific workouts, times, and distances. You can't let each other down because you know your buddy is counting on you – and you are a little bit afraid he might get into better shape than you if he does the workout while you take a rest day.

I Need a Run Buddy – This buddy is willing to go for a run at the drop of a hat. She is also a good ear, and that's why you need her at the drop of a hat. She can help you burn some steam and regroup when you are feeling stressed.

I Will if You Will Buddy – This buddy helps you talk yourself into going for a run. I might text her and ask,

"Are you running today?" Her reply makes me commit. "Sure, what time do you want to go?" My commitment to her is the same. If she texts me with a similar question, we run.

I Miss My Buddy Buddy – This is the friend that you have grown to love over miles and miles. You haven't seen her for a time and a run is the perfect way to catch up. You may not have expected to grow to love her so much, but the shared dreams and discouragements, not to mention the misery over those long miles, have cemented your friendship.

I'm just a Runner Buddy – This buddy isn't one of your regular workout partners, but he is a runner, so you are friends. That's how it works – runners feel kinship to runners. You might only run together once or twice a year, but when the regular buddies are not available you can find a friend to tag along.

Running buddies come in many shapes, sizes, ages, and genders. Some running buddies never go for a run together, but they enjoy talking about running when they are together. This much I know … If you become a runner, your social circles will expand in ways you never anticipated. Running will enrich your social life – it did that for mine!

Try this:

Invite a friend to take up running along with you or be courageous and ask a runner you know if you can tag along on his next run. Mention on social media that you are going for a run and see who will ask to join you. Your circle of friends will begin to grow as other runners learn that you have joined the ranks of happy runners.

Take a Rest

Believe it or not, athletes and those who want to be athletes can benefit from taking a rest. In fact, training plans for any race length from 5K to marathon incorporate rest days into the training schedule. Rest days allow your body to recuperate from the challenges of a training schedule. I have found that even a short break or rest during a run can sometimes help me run farther.

Take a rest to catch your breath. A beginning runner, or even an experienced runner adding distance to her routine, can benefit from a short walk break. For beginners, a walk break is a chance to catch your breath and discover that you can soon recover and run a little farther. Use these breaks to push yourself that extra half mile. Next time you run, shorten the break while covering the same distance.

Take a rest to rejuvenate your muscles. It's okay to give your legs and lungs a day off. In fact, rest days may help to prevent injury, especially stress injuries. Most training schedules incorporate one or two rest days into weekly training. If the schedule says to take time off – do it.

Take a rest to give your brain a break. I have found that rest days are as important to my mental commitment as they are to my physical well-being. When I take some time off, I miss running. Missing something, at least for me, makes it more appealing. I miss the feeling of accomplishment I get after a good run. I miss the feeling of physical exhaustion and the relaxation of recovery. I miss fresh air surging through my lungs into my veins to fuel my brain. I miss my running buddies and I have a renewed desire to go for a run.

Take a rest to prevent injury. In my book, *The Hard Run: Painful Lessons from a Running Granny*, I discuss the need to recognize warning signs indicating that we are doing harm to ourselves. Ignoring those signs as they relate to running can lead to stress injuries that sideline a runner longer than needed. Too many miles too many days in a row can undermine your best intentions.

*Discomfort that does not subside with rest is an indication that you have an injury that may need treatment from a healthcare professional.

Try this:

Commit to run three to four days per week adding mileage gradually. On days you don't run, do another enjoyable physical activity. It's called "cross training" and we will discuss it in a later chapter. Be sure to make at least one of those days a true rest day. Our Creator rested one day of the week and so should you.

Time to Commit

If you have been reading this book and implementing the lessons in the previous chapters then you've conquered your pride, your fear, and your worries over what to wear. Maybe you found a buddy to run with you or you put together an awesome playlist. You've logged a few miles, but the weather keeps you indoors some days, or your busy schedule prevents a run on other days. You might even be a little sore from time to time. You could be tempted to take more rest days than you really need. How are you going to stay committed to this new adventure we call "running?"

One of the best ways to stay committed is to register for a race.

Of course, there is always this excuse. "Oh, but I've just begun and I am not fast enough to run a race." Yeah, we've all thought that.

I've got some news for you ...

Nobody cares if you are not fast. They are just glad you are participating. Runners are cool like that – they want everyone to share in the fun. Remember that little worry you have about not being fast enough? It will motivate you to push yourself.

Then there is this excuse, "I don't think I can run 3.1 miles."

I'll let you in on a little secret, most races are "Fun Runs." You can walk if you need! However, if you register and follow a training plan, you'll be able to run 3.1 miles just fine.

Your friends and family may ask, "Why would anyone *pay* to run?"

Paid registration will keep you running on a regular basis. There is something strangely motivating about the financial obligation of a race fee and someone, even a faceless race director, knowing that you are planning to participate.

Try this:

Find a local fun run in which to participate. Small town races are usually relaxed and the registration fees are not as pricey as more recognizable, nationally known races. Many areas have 5K races themed around holidays such as Independence Day, Thanksgiving, Christmas, and New Year's Day. If you have guilty feelings about spending the money, find a race that benefits a cause such as a local food drive or homeless shelter. Then run and enjoy your first race. You'll be glad you did.

Follow a Plan

Congratulations, you have committed to a race! Do you know how to prepare for one? You might be surprised to learn that the answer is NOT to try to run farther and faster every day. A good training plan will include short runs, long runs, speed work, and cross training/rest days.

What is the best training plan? That depends on the runner.

First, it must be customized for you. It will take into consideration your current running routine such as weekly mileage, pace, and the date of the race for which you are preparing.

Second, it must be user friendly for the runner. I like to cross things off a list. My satisfaction is visual, so a plan that I can find online, plug in my stats and print out is perfect. Other runners like digital reminders. A phone app such as MapMyRun or Runkeeper that has a coaching option works for best them. Couch to 5K is a standardized schedule for new runners. The runner chooses whether to run for time or for distance. Couch to

5K can be found in book form, but it also has the convenience of a mobile app.

Third, it must have variety. Long runs build stamina. Speed work improves pace. Cross training builds strength and injury prevention. Short runs help muscles recover from long runs. Rest days? We talked about their value in a previous chapter. Varying running workouts tricks the brain and aids in maintaining commitment to the plan.

Fourth, it must be forgiving. Don't pick a training program so intense that forced time off due to illness or family obligations discourages you from completing the goal. If it adds mileage too quickly or quickens the pace too soon, it will be difficult to continue through challenges and may result in discouragement and abandonment of the race goal. Remember, the purpose of the race commitment and training plan is to develop a habit of consistent running.

Try this:

Time a mile or two on your next run then search online for a training plan you can begin six to nine weeks prior to your first fun run. Plug in your timed pace, race distance, and race date to generate a training plan customized for you. Do your best to follow the outlined workouts and don't quit if you have a small setback. Do your best. This will be your first race and you will have opportunities to not only better prepare, but to perform better in future races.

Carol M Green

Section II

Mental Trickery

Visit with any runner and she will tell you that a large part of running is in your head. This section of the book will give you tricks and ideas to help you endure when your brain says, "Quit!" That doesn't mean your legs and lungs aren't going to want to betray you at times, but the mental tricks will help you outsmart your rebelling body parts.

Try different mental tricks to discover those that work best for you. You may even come up with some of your own.

Wear Running Clothes

Runners don't always want to run. I will admit that I don't feel like running every morning when I get out of bed. In fact, I often lie there thinking of ways to get out of running that day. I have too much to do. It's cold outside. I ran yesterday. I don't have any running buddies to keep me company today. The longer I lie there, the longer the list!

I have learned this one simple trick. If I get up and don my running clothes, shoes included, something magical often happens. My brain recognizes that I am a runner. My clothes make me look and feel like a runner. (Refer to What Will You Wear? at the beginning of this book.) It doesn't always happen immediately and I think that is why it works. I am convinced that I don't have to run as I lace up my shoes. While my lazier self is still rationalizing a non-run day, the feel of my running clothes is gently reminding me that I am a runner and I will feel better after I have logged a few miles. It can take all day before I actually get out the door, but rarely do I miss a run if I have first chosen to dress the part.

Runners who choose to get up before the sun may want to sleep in their sports bra, tights, and wicking shirt.

When the alarm goes off and the eyes fly open, the self-talk can be, "Oh, I'm dressed! I must be going for a run."

Runners who work a nine to five job and do most of their running in the evening can change into running gear as soon as possible after work.

I have long said, "Looking good is half the battle." That usually refers to a public speaking assignment or scholarship or job interview, but it holds true with running as well. If you are struggling to log miles, get out of bed, wear your running clothes, shoes included, and you might find that you truly are a runner!

Try this:

Lay your gear out at night before you retire for the evening. In the morning, throw the running clothes on before breakfast. That might be all it takes. If not, let the magic have time to work. After you've completed a few tasks around the house, the open road may be calling. If you plan to run in the evening, don your running outfit as early as possible. Give it a try and see how effective this simple trick can be.

Turn a Corner

The temptation to stop during a run, especially when unaccompanied by a buddy, can arise at any time. This struggle seems more common during casual runs than when following a training plan. I use the following mental trick to keep me moving when I want to quit. I've taught it to my middle school cross country runners and it works for them, too.

When on a run choose a landmark and plan to run to that mark before taking a walking break. Give yourself permission to rest when you reach the goal. It may be a crossroad or a driveway or mailbox. Rural running offers fields, canals and ditch banks, even tractors parked in fields that can be used for landmarks. Track running offers hundred, two hundred, and four hundred meter marks that can be used for distance goals. Measuring distance or time on a treadmill can serve as landmarks as well.

Once you have reached the goal, force yourself to run beyond the landmark – even if it's only a few steps. If the goal is a crossroads or corner, run around the corner. It can be as short as ten steps around the corner or beyond the goal. You will often discover that you can keep going because you have endured through the difficult part of the run. Perhaps the scenery has changed or even better, you've encountered a small descent and the terrain is easier to negotiate. You may want to keep going.

This trick can be used at the end of a run, or several times during the workout. Anytime the goal is attained, choose to take ten more steps, pass one more power pole, or reach one more driveway.

This mental trick can help you in other parts of your life. If you think you can't keep going, find a point to rest and then physically or figuratively turn a corner. Hang in there a little longer than you thought you could. Things might get easier!

Try this:

Go for a casual run. Determine how far you will go before taking a walk break or ending your run. When you reach that point, don't stop! Take a few more strides, then you can rest. However, if rest is not needed because your perspective has changed, choose another stopping point farther down the path. When you reach that point, apply this technique and take a few more strides!

Cover New Ground

A change of perspective can enhance the experience of a regular run. My regular running buddy and I were recently joined by another friend. Our route was unfamiliar to her and she commented that it kind of made the running easier because she didn't know where she was going. She was just running. Covering new ground can make a difference whether that new ground is a physical location or simply a new running experience.

A change of location can make your run more interesting and tolerable. During my night run of the Grand Teton Relay 2014, I was all alone. It was dark and the course was off road, so I had no familiar landmarks. This was the first time I had experienced a night run all by myself. A few glow sticks were placed along the path, but they were easy to overlook. I forgot to start my run clock and had no idea how much terrain I had covered until a volunteer shouted, "Turn here!" I paused, removed my headphones and asked, "How far?" I thought I had another half mile. When he told me I only had 100 feet to go I sprinted gleefully to the end! I was surprised and happy that my night run was over.

Cover new ground or change your perspective in any number of ways. Run your usual route backwards. Head out the door at a different time of day. Don't forget to wear reflective clothing if you are going for a night run – and take a buddy along. Break in a new running buddy, or encourage a friend to go for her first run. The latter will help you see how far you've come since your own first run. Run in the rain. Using a mobile app, draw a figure or write a word with your route. You'll be so focused on the drawing that the workout will be over before you know it.

Try this:

Change things up on your very next run. Implement one idea from the list above. After your workout, evaluate what a change of perspective did or did not do for you. You might be surprised how much you can do when you don't really know what you are doing.

Read Something Inspiring

Time spent away from running can be as important as time spent on the run. That is why I suggest you read something inspiring. I'm not talking about a fortune cookie, or a subway print found on Pinterest, or even this book – although I am grateful you are reading it and I hope it helps. I'm talking about reading a book that inspires you and leaves you wanting to do and be more.

My daughter sent me a message to tell me her six-year-old can read *Green Eggs and Ham* by Dr. Seuss. It's one of my favorites, 1) because it is challenging and entertaining to read aloud, and 2) its message is to try new things. I love to read it to my grandchildren and now they can begin to read it to me.

I once read *Mary Kay* by Mary Kay Ash, the founder of Mary Kay Cosmetics. It left me feeling encouraged and capable.

When I was in the fourth grade, I read *The Hobbit* for the first time. J.R.R. Tolkien brought my nightmares to life and taught me that everyone has talent and purpose. I haven't read it as many times as I've *read Green Eggs and Ham* or my favorite book of scripture, but *The*

Hobbit is a book that inspires me each time I explore its pages.

Running the Edge by Tim Catalano and Adam Goucher, was recommended to me by a friend, a cousin of one of the authors. It taught me new things about running; things that I had not already discovered on my own.

Try this:

If your desire to run is waning ... read something running related such as a runner's biography or a classic running novel. Suggestions:

> *Running with the Buffaloes* by Chris Lear
> *Unbroken* by Laura Hillenbrand
> *Run to Overcome* by Meb Keflezighi, Dick Patrick, and Joan Benoit Samuelson

If you've been injured and need some down time to recover ... read something entertaining to pass the time or something that will instill patience and positivity. Suggestions:

> *The Power of Positive Thinking* by Dr. Norman Vincent Peale
> *Gone With the Wind* by Margaret Mitchell
> *Running the Edge* by Tim Catalano and Adam Goucher

If your improvement is slow and you need daily motivation ... read something that inspires you daily such as your favorite book of scripture, a daily motivational tip from a life coach, or browse a recent copy of a running magazine.

Remember, running is hard. Life is hard. It's going to take a little help to get you through it. Reading something that inspires, uplifts, or encourages doing one's best can keep you on the running path both mentally and physically. You can read and learn from those who have gone before. It might make things a little bit easier.

Log Your Workout

One of my favorite training tools is a record, or log, of my running workout. Whether you are tracking miles, reps, or time in the gym, you will find great satisfaction in watching the numbers add up each month. As your running journal grows, you will find ways to challenge yourself. Perhaps you find that the two days you ran last week can be increased to three days this week, or even four. If your miles were good one week, you may think to yourself, "I can add a mile here and a mile there to stay consistent or even surpass last week's mileage."

There are many ways to log your efforts from writing miles on a wall calendar to using an app that gives added information such as pace and calories burned. Here are just a few.

Calendar

You choose the information you want to record. Are you adding up miles each month or do you simply want to cross off each day in an effort to obtain consistency? A wall calendar is public and allows family members or co-workers to see your progress which will hold you accountable and encourage you along the way.

Step Trackers

These tools can be as simple as a clip-on pedometer or as advanced as a smart watch that syncs with your phone. If you carry your smart phone on your person most of the time, download an app that counts steps on your phone. Remember, these tools will record total steps and may not give the best running feedback. For instance, if the device is not equipped with GPS functionality, your longer running strides may report with less mileage than you travelled. This may not be important if you are using the device to record and compare day to day movement.

Fitness Apps

A fitness app will provide more information than a step tracker. It can track your workout, provide workout analytics, link your favorite music, and even give feedback during the workout. I like Map My Run. I set mine to give feedback every half mile. It tells me how far and how fast (or slow) I am going. You can even share the information on Facebook – if you are brave enough!

Follow a Training Plan

If you are goal minded and have decided to train for a 5K or longer, download a training plan and then write all over it. Record your distance and time. You might even add some insights about the workout such as, "Today's run was hard." Or, "I rocked it today! Fifteen seconds under goal pace!" And so on.

Report to Friends

I belong to a group of family and friends that record our miles and share them with each other. This can help keep you on task. "They are expecting me to log something today. I better get out the door." Or, "If I just go two more miles, I will have the most miles in the group!" Including others in your fitness pursuits helps encourage everyone to reach their goals. Never underestimate the value of friends!

Try this:

If you are having trouble with consistency in your training routine, maybe it's time to find a new way to keep you accountable. Logging your workouts and possibly sharing them with others can keep you motivated.

Begin with a simple calendar or notebook. You can create a log on a spreadsheet if that is in your skill set. Keep a log for a few days, then review it and record your thoughts about the information you have kept.

If you have a running friend, text him or her about your rainy run, your slow run, or your new personal record.

Download a tracking app and learn to use it. You can share the information with the world on social media, keep it private, or delete it altogether!

If you have been logging your workout and need motivation, try something different or a combination of those listed above. The best training log (and yes, I get asked this question) is the one that works for you, just like the best running shoe is the one that fits you best.

Carol M Green

Share the Love

Sharing the love, or sharing your running workout, might seem a little narcissistic, but it can also be an act of service. We will get to that, but first, let's look at ways it can help you.

The previous chapter discusses methods of logging your workout and why that helps. Think of logging the workout as recording a goal. A goal written down is firmer than one simply floating about in your head. In fact, a goal not written, is probably only an idea. Compare sharing your workout to sharing a written goal with others. Sharing goals tends to make the goal setter more accountable and determined to reach the goal. Sharing what you have already accomplished, or your workout, will also make you more accountable and determined to continue.

Anticipation of sharing your workout might make you run longer, faster, or more frequently. Perhaps you will even be motivated to run on days that are less than pleasant, such as, windy, rainy, or particularly busy days. All those things are positive effects of sharing the running love.

Some of us are motivated by our positive influence on others. If you are a giver, a server, or an encourager of your fellow man, woman or child, you may be more inclined to share your experiences to improve the lives of others. Let's look at ways your sharing can be a service.

To Your Running Buddy

I promise that your running buddy needs some motivation from time to time, just like you. I have received a text from a friend telling me about her run and, whether through guilt or envy, I have been motivated to lace up and hit the road. Her text served as an encouragement to me.

To Your Family

Stop viewing exercise and good health as self-serving. You owe it to those people whom you love to take care of yourself. They are many – your spouse, your children, your grandchildren, your church, and even your friends and community. If you are healthy, you can better serve them in all ways. As they see you taking care of your health, they may also feel invited to take care of their physical well-being.

To Your Observers

These are your friends and acquaintances that watch you from afar. In other words, they are those who would like to run, but will not voice it because they, like you once did, are concerned about those things we discussed in the first chapters of this book. They might be afraid of the judgements of others if they take up running. The judgements aren't critiques so much as they are admiration or envy. Your observers are those who have not yet conquered their fear of discomfort, failure or the unknown that looms before them. Your observers are watching to see if you can be successful, because if you can do it, perhaps they can do it as well. They may be watching you from afar, but they may be your best friend or your neighbor. Invite them to join you.

To Discouraged Runners

Yes, it happens from time to time. Runners get discouraged, often from things that sideline them such as an injury, illness, change of seasons, or schedule changes. It's okay to share a workout that says, "It wasn't pretty and it wasn't far, but I went for a run." It's okay to share that you are discouraged because you haven't been able to run due to one of those reasons. It is especially important and encouraging to share when you have conquered the setback and you are back in the running mode.

Try this:

You can share your workout log, your workout thoughts and feelings, or a photo in many ways. Sharing can be as targeted as a text to a running buddy or as broad as a photo shared on a social running page. Do what works for you.

Message a friend through a phone text, email or social media. "I ran 2 miles today! That's a record for me!" or, "I'll run if you will." How about, "I was slow today, but I did it!"

Post a screen shot of your running app feedback complete with distance, pace, and course map. This one takes courage because it is available to the world! You might be surprised at the positive comments you receive. Nobody ever posts, "You idiot! Can't you run any faster than that? How lazy can you get?" Nope. Nobody does that.

Even more courageous is a picture of your red sweaty post run face. That's honesty for you!

If you have a blog, write about your running experiences. Who knows, blogging may be inspire you to write a book of encouragement for other runners.

Don't forget to tell the world how much running has improved your life, because I promise, it will.

Chew Some Gum

This mental trick might not sound like much of a tip. It may sound too simple or even too dangerous for some. In fact, I was skeptical and had been running for quite some time before trying it. When other runners mentioned that they couldn't get along without chewing gum on the run, I thought they were crazy. I was convinced that having a piece of gum in my mouth would present a choking hazard while I was gasping for precious breaths of air! I don't remember why I finally decided to give chewing gum on the run a try, but I'm glad I did.

Chewing a piece of gum provides a distraction for your brain. Who doesn't need to think about something other than the fact that they are breathing hard, their legs are tired and they would like to stop for a break and a drink of water?

Like the mind trick discussed in a previous chapter, *Wear Your Running Clothes,* a stick of gum in your mouth can tell your brain it is time to run, especially if you chew the same flavor on most of your runs. I prefer peppermint, but any gum is better than no gum at all! If you are not typically a gum chewer, save it only for running. The "it's time to run" effect will be all the stronger as your brain associates the gum with running.

The rhythm of chewing helps you settle into a running rhythm. Maintaining a running rhythm can help you stay on the road longer, thus allowing you to log more miles. Logging more miles improves your fitness and might also make it fun to report to your running friends! (See previous chapter – Log Your Workout)

In warm and hot temperatures, it can be tempting to stop for a drink of water. If you have hydrated properly, your body isn't so much in need of the drink as is your brain. Although a dry mouth might feel uncomfortable, it is your muscles that need the fluid. We will discuss hydration further in an upcoming chapter. For comfort, a stick of chewing gum is the next best thing to a drink of water. It will keep your mouth lubricated and lessen the discomfort of a warm weather run.

Gum tastes good. A fresh piece of gum tastes even better. If you plan to be on the road, trail, or treadmill longer than 45 minutes, stash a stick in your pocket or running belt. If the run gets to feel monotonous or your current stick of gum loses its appeal, switch it out for a fresh one. If you have become accustomed to popping a piece of gum in your mouth prior to your run, your brain may be tricked into thinking you are just getting started and the second half of that long run might not feel so intimidating.

Try this:

Obtain two or three flavors of chewing gum to try out during the next few weeks. Minty flavors will be the most refreshing during warm weather, however, they can be truly brisk during cooler temps. You might want to opt for cinnamon or another mild flavor on cold days.

When you find a flavor that suits you, don't start your run without it. If you are having a hard time getting out the door because you simply don't feel like running today, pop a stick of your running gum in your mouth, lace up your shoes, turn on your logging device and step outside. You'll be on the run before you know it.

Find a Cause

Running for a cause different from your own physical and mental well-being adds more purpose to your new hobby. Anything done with purpose adds greater degrees of dedication. Finding a cause to which you can commit will help you keep logging miles.

If you have been running for a while you may find that you are suddenly interested in a variety of causes, perhaps even some you had not considered previously. This could be that you have been bitten by the racing bug and have discovered that many fun runs benefit cancer research, food banks, and other community projects. There are two local fun runs held annually in my small community. We won't count the Turkey Trot on Thanksgiving Day, as it is simply for a group of friends trying to get ahead of the holiday's indulgence while the turkey and stuffing roasts in the oven! The other two are for causes that I have managed to get behind. One benefits the schools' cross country teams and the other benefits our local food bank. I am a co-organizer, supporter, and promoter of both. Sometimes I participate and sometimes I facilitate. Either way, these races keep me honest as those present know that I profess to be a runner. I have to back it up!

Is there a way you can volunteer as a runner? As the school's cross country program began to grow it became obvious that the coach needed some help, if only for crowd control. I offered my support and soon found that I was committed to running nearly every weekday afternoon during the fall season. As I grew to know the athletes and watched them grow as runners, my commitment to the program grew stronger. I have been there several years and now have an official coaching position with a team. Cross country has become one of my causes.

Try this:

Consider some things that give you cause for concern. Are you anxious about diseases such as cancer or multiple sclerosis? There are races that support research for those diseases. Homelessness? Childhood hunger? Chances are you can find a local race that raises funds to support these causes. Do an online search to locate one that will motivate you to participate. Then register and begin training. Don't forget to tell your friends and family that you have made the commitment.

Make it Musical

This mental trick will help you add time to your running workout. Music is a nice mental diversion when you are logging miles on the run, especially if you are running alone. You can use it to extend the length of your workout. Whether your goal is to log more miles or burn more calories, music can help you make it happen.

How does it work?

Music keeps your mind off your discomfort – at least it helps. When you are listening to music the sound of your own breathing is softened. If you are like me, the sound of your lungs pulling air in and pushing it out can send off a mental alarm. Softening the sound can keep the "I'm working too hard" and "I want to quit" thoughts at bay. While music can be a time waster of sorts, wasting time is a good thing while on the run as it allows you to get lost in the words and rhythms. Before you know it, you have covered a few hundred meters while listening to your favorite song. The rhythm, or beat, also aids in finding a consistent pace. Just as chewing a stick of gum will help you settle into a pace, your steps will automatically sync with the music often without your even noticing it. This is great unless your favorite song is a crooning ballad. Be sure to choose something with a good tempo to keep you moving along. If the tempo is too slow, it will feel sluggish and your brain may think, "I feel like a snail." Nobody wants to feel like a snail.

Try this:

Create a playlist of songs you often find yourself singing aloud. They should be upbeat enough to keep you moving, but not so fast that you get exhausted trying to keep up with the beat. If you can sing all the words to the song while running, the beat is too slow. If you can't belt out any phrases while on the run, find something a little slower.

Check the time length and number of songs on your playlist. If you typically run for 30 minutes, make sure your playlist lasts longer than that. Add 10 to 15 minutes for every mile you want to log. You can use the shuffle and repeat modes to extend the playlist if you prefer. However, if you happen to hear a song for a second time it may trick you into thinking your workout is completed and you may be tempted to stop.

Run until you have heard the playlist once through. A variation would be to run until you have heard your favorite song play twice.

To avoid monotony, update your playlist from time to time to keep your experience fresh.

Whether you are a beginning runner or a seasoned competitor, you can benefit by changing up your running playlist to trick you into running longer. You can use this mental trick to help you endure other tasks like mowing the yard, painting a room, or canning vegetables!

Run Farther

Adding distance at the beginning of your run is a mental trick that can be more effective than simply running farther. It is especially helpful when training for a 10K or half marathon. Those long runs can feel daunting as they increase in distance each week, especially when you are training for your first long race. I learned this while training for a half marathon. As the workouts increased in length, I began adding mileage at the beginning of a familiar course. Although the distance was farther, I found that keeping the last few miles consistent made the end of the run feel like any other run.

Here is the mental trick.

Adding mileage or distance at the beginning of a run allows the runner to finish on familiar territory. The last mile of a four-mile run will feel familiar and conquerable as it is the same mile he usually runs at the end of a three-mile run. The runner will think, "I've got one mile to go. I've got this." Simply adding distance at the end of a route with which he is familiar may have the opposite effect. The runner will be mentally ready to quit prior to the added distance for the same reasons - he is on the last mile of his usual route and the thought of going one more mile may be overwhelming. Although the distance is the same in both situations, an additional mile will be more mentally challenging when added at the end of the familiar route than if it is tackled at the beginning.

Try this:

Run a familiar route on Monday and again on Wednesday. On Friday or Saturday run the same route, but add a half mile or more prior to tackling the same Monday/Wednesday route.

If you typically begin your run from your front door, try running a loop around your neighborhood before following your regular route. If you begin your run near a park or high school track, do a couple laps on the track or walking path before heading out on a road course. I guarantee it will help make the longer distance feel easier than trying to tackle it at the end of the run.

The idea of longer distance may be challenging at the beginning of your workout, but by the end when you are on familiar territory it will feel conquerable. Follow this same practice for a few weeks and soon you will have doubled the distance on your long runs. Your next 5K race will feel short and fast because you have been covering greater distance. It's all about perspective!

Whether you are a beginning runner or a seasoned competitor, this mental trick can help you in other parts of your life. When faced with a new challenge, surround yourself with familiarity. The people, positive practices and places that have helped you achieve success in the past can help you conquer the challenges ahead.

Section III

Trouble Shooting

There are sure to be troubles along your path. This section of the book discusses ways to overcome those setbacks or shoot down your troubles. Injuries, life events, mental fatigue, and other factors beyond your control may seem to derail you from time to time. Be patient with these setbacks.

Remember, you can always start over. You have the tools and know what it takes to begin – again.

Hydration is Key

There is much information available about hydration and exercise. Some of it is helpful and some is very confusing. What we do know is that you need to drink enough water. There isn't a One-Size-Fits-All measurement. However, the traditional 64 ounces of water per day is a good place to begin. Your hydration needs will vary with the weather and your level of exercise. For instance, I know that if I am hydrated I can do a six-mile run without stopping for water. If the weather is particularly warm I may feel as if I need something mid-run. I can choose to stop for a drink, tough it out, or chew some gum. However, if I don't re-hydrate mid-run or post-run, I will have cramping and muscle soreness later.

Thirst is a good indicator that you need to drink something, but it may take some time to learn how much water YOU need and when it is most beneficial for you.

Muscle cramping can also be caused by dehydration. Although there may be other factors to this kind of discomfort, drinking water is a quick diagnostic and simple way to alleviate muscle problems due to dehydration.

Other indications that you need a drink of water are fatigue, light headedness, and headaches.

Try this:

If you plan to go for a morning run, be sure to drink 8 – 16 ounces of water late in the evening. I know, I know, but getting out of bed once in the night is far better than cramping during a run or throughout the day.

If you have difficulty exercising after having downed a glass of water, be sure to drink 4 – 8 ounces at least one hour prior to your run, even if you downed the suggested fluid the evening before.

In hot weather, either carry water with you, or stash a water bottle somewhere along your route prior to your workout and take a water break mid-run.

Always hydrate post-run. Always.

Two things to remember …

1 - Water is your best option for hydration. Sports drinks and chocolate milk are fine, but not necessary for success. Water is usually cheaper and more readily available.

2 – It is possible to over hydrate, but you probably won't. It is very difficult to over hydrate, so when in doubt, drink it up!

Cool it Down

Neglecting to cool down and stretch can lead to muscle cramps and tenderness which can, in turn, lead to stress injuries and muscle tears. I learned this lesson the hard way and was forced to take time off. Do as I say, not as I did!

Unfortunately, it is very tempting and easy to overlook this simple practice, especially after a race or a particularly difficult workout. At the end of my first 5K, as I expect it is with many runners, all I wanted was the water bottle offered and to collapse on the grass in a heap. It was all I could do to stand while the race volunteer removed my racing chip from my ankle and then keep moving out of the way of other finishers. I was exhausted for the rest of the day and very sore for several days to follow.

While it is normal to be sore after a race, the pain will be lessened if you take time to do what I call "walk it out" before treating yourself to a day of lazing around. This holds true for your day to day running workouts as well. Don't collapse in a heap. Take time to walk followed by a few minutes of stretching.

Why is stretching important? Did you read the fifth chapter of this book, Learn to Stretch? It's all there and even though you may be getting better at this running thing, the rules still apply. Stretching after a workout will aid in injury prevention, loosen tight muscles, increase flexibility and balance, aid in relaxation, and give you time to reflect on whatever you may need to ponder – your run, your goals, your life in general, the cobweb in the corner. You name it. If it needs reflecting upon, it will appear much clearer after your run than before.

Try this:

Map out a route that begins and ends a few hundred meters away from your front door. You can use the distance to warm up, start your running app, determine if your shoes are laced up just right, and gather your courage if needed. Most importantly, this will provide a natural cool down route as you return home for a few minutes of stretching. I prefer about a half mile (800 meters) warm up and cool down. I can almost feel my calf muscles relax at about 750 meters from my home!

You can stretch indoors or outdoors. In warm weather, a soft carpet of grass can be especially relaxing. Use your front step to do some simple calf raises and drops. Step up on the step with one foot and bend into your knee to stretch your hamstrings and glutes. Do some standing figure four stretches or yoga pigeon pose to keep your sciatic nerve from screaming at you. Down dog and cobra will loosen your lower back. Be sure to stretch out all your major muscle groups.

Caution: Over stretching can aggravate stressed tendons and even pull tight muscles. Stretch when your muscles are warm and go slow and easy.

Remember, this is a time to relax and reflect. Don't overlook the cool down and stretching phase of your workout!

Carol M Green

Examine Your Soles

In the first section of this book we talked about what to wear. Hopefully, you followed the instructions and obtained a good pair of running shoes. Unfortunately, shoes won't last forever. You should get a few hundred miles out of them, but keep an eye on your sole so you know when to replace them.

If you are having lower leg, foot or ankle troubles, examine the tread wear on the bottom of your running shoes. It can tell you a lot.

I had been struggling with Achilles tendonitis for some time. I felt impressed to look at the wear patterns on my shoes. They indicated that I was heel striking with my left foot – pounding away at an already inflamed Achilles tendon. The tread on the heel of my left shoe had been worn smooth. This wear pattern showed me that I needed to change my gait or run a little lighter so I could land on the middle of my foot. After making a conscious effort to correct my gait, the tendonitis began to improve.

There are many things you can learn by examining the soles of your running shoes. Ideally, the wear pattern should be generalized with more wear in the middle of the shoe. If it is uneven you may need to make corrections in your form.

Try this:

Hold your shoes side by side with the soles facing you, arches together. Look for generalized wear vs. wear in one area such as the heel or outside edge.

Is there wear on the heels or toes? Perhaps you need to pick up your feet and step lighter.

The wear patterns should be similar on both shoes. If not, what can you see? Are you favoring one leg or dragging one foot?

Do you need a different style of running shoe? You may need help with this decision. Take your worn shoes to a running store and have them help you discover which shoe is best for you. It's worth the time and investment.

Is it time for new shoes? Are you experiencing new discomfort in your feet or lower legs? If you have worn through any layers of the sole, whether in one spot or with a general wear pattern, you are past due. Go get some new shoes!

The right pair of shoes in good condition coupled with proper form will help to keep you running and injury free.

Massage Tired Muscles

If you've been running for a few weeks, chances are you've had to deal with some aches and pains. Massage therapy could be the answer.

I had been diligently doing my best to treat a nagging case of Sciatica (mine) with stretching, Ibuprofen, ointments, rest, and clam shell exercises. It wasn't improving so I decided to call in the big guns and have my first legitimate therapeutic massage.

I had long been leery of massage, mostly because I am ticklish. I even bypassed the free foot massages at the finish line of some of my favorite races – until the Grand Teton Relay 2014. My teammate coerced me and I succumbed. I was immediately fond of the lady working on my ankles and feet. I would have brought her home if I could.

That convinced me to seek help from a massage therapist. I had my first therapeutic massage and there was not any giggling going on! Her elbow jammed into my left hip. My heel touched my derriere. The massage oil smelled like a medicine cabinet belonging to a geriatric. I had to go to my happy place a time or two. It hurt so good!

I am happy to report that the massage alleviated the pain. She told me she could fix it and she did. I think I am a believer.

You may be experiencing some discomfort and need the aid of a massage therapist, or you might benefit from learning to use a tennis ball to massage the kinks away. You could be surprised at the many uses of these brightly colored orbs. They're not just for tennis players anymore!

Try this:

A tennis ball fits under your foot and can be used to massage from heel to toe while sitting in a chair. You can throw it in your purse or bag and take it with you to work, the doctor's office, library, and even at work or on an airplane. Use it anywhere you will be sitting for a length of time.

A tennis ball can isolate sore spots in the upper calf. Sit on the floor and roll it around under your leg. You will know the spot when you find it by the surprising tenderness you had not noticed previously. Take some deep breaths while you continue to keep pressure on the sore spot until it releases. Roll the ball around as you are likely to find another area on the same calf that is tight.

Try the same technique on your hamstrings. It works for them, too.

While sitting on the floor, place the tennis ball between your quadricep muscle and the palm of your hand. Use your palm to roll the ball around, massaging the entire quadricep until it feels relaxed.

Bye, bye, Sciatica! Position the tennis ball under your left or right Gluteus Maximus and roll around until you find the sore spot. You'll know it when have a sudden gasp for air! Hold that position until you feel the muscle relax. Your Sciatic nerve will thank you.

There are many varieties of massage sticks and foam rollers on the market for athletes. If you find massage works for you, you may want to invest in some. In the meantime, pick up a tennis ball. Tennis balls are convenient and inexpensive. You can pack them in your purse, pocket, or gym bag.

Don't let those aches and pains go for too long. If you don't find relief quickly with your home remedies, seek help from someone who knows more than you. Your family physician, massage therapists, and even the pros at your favorite running store should be able to help. Try a tennis ball first. You don't have to wait for an appointment and you can afford it.

Carol M Green

Change it Up

Runners are often convinced that we are especially tough because we can run miles and miles. While it is true that our legs and lungs are in great condition there are parts of our physique that often get neglected. Cross training can be especially helpful in strengthening those neglected parts.

It isn't only that we think we are tough, but most runners would rather take their training outside than indoors. Taking your workout outdoors can make it difficult to implement weight training and other cross training activities into workouts.

Cross training can be any physical activity that differs from your regular workout routine. Strength training is one type of cross training for runners, while running is a form of cross training for wrestlers, football players, or anyone trying to increase endurance for their favorite activity. Running makes me a better skier and biking makes me a better runner.

Strength training can go a long way in injury prevention and improved performance. You don't have to invest a lot of time to gain those added benefits. That's nice, because we all know you would rather be outdoors logging miles.

Engaging in varied physical activities breaks up the monotony of your sport. No matter how much you love your sport, you can benefit from a change of pace, both physically and mentally.

Cross training can strengthen neglected body parts. Runners often develop weak Gluteus Maximus muscles. This can result in discomfort as the Sciatic nerve can be pinched and lead to pain in the hip and leg. A little strength training and yoga can help prevent or alleviate this issue.

Cross training can expand your social circles. I love my running buddies, but if I only run, then my workout friends are limited to those few friends who run. (I'm trying to expand the running circles!) Biking, swimming, and tennis can broaden your social community as you engage with these enthusiastic athletes.

Cross training can remind you why you love your sport. If you find yourself in a rut or dreading your run, take a few days off and do a different physical activity. You may find that you are missing your running workout, the very one that you had been dreading.

Try this:

Choose one or two days a week to do something different, even if it only lasts a half hour. You can visit the gym and attend a yoga class or do some light upper body weight training.

Go for a swim. This is not a dip or a soak in a hot tub, but an actual lap swim to work your upper body – arms, shoulders and back. Swimming laps will provide a good cardio workout and loosen up those tired legs as well.

Call a friend and go for a bike ride. Play tennis, ping pong, volleyball or basketball. Any activity that keeps you moving is good for the body and good for the soul.

The goal is to stay healthy and keep running. Cross training can help make that happen.

Take Time Off

In the first section of this book we discussed incorporating rest days into your regular running routine to prevent injury and keep you motivated. What if the unfortunate happens and you become injured? You may need to take a little more time away from running. If this happens, refer to the previous chapter for ways you can stay active while recuperating from a running injury.

While I am an advocate of enduring pain and discomfort when the body and mind can benefit from the challenge, I also know there is wisdom in caution. The tricky part is discerning when to go and when to stop during a workout or training plan. I wrote an entire book about recognizing what kind of discomfort you are experiencing, but this discussion deals with knowing when to take time off.

I began following a training plan early one year to help me be more consistent in my running. Unfortunately, the weather in Idaho in January is not consistent. The only consistent thing in Idaho's weather is change. I postponed a run on a warm sunny day because I was extra busy and knew I would have more time the next day. To my dismay, the following day was dumping heavy wet snow! I have endured snowy runs in the past.

In fact, I quite enjoy them. However, I spent the previous summer with an injury that nagged me for six months, so I decided not to risk another injury on the slick and snowy roads.

Injuries can happen to runners. Most often they manifest themselves in the form of stress related problems such as tendonitis, plantar fasciitis and even muscle tears. However, the occasional rolled ankle or dog bite can occur. Avoid rolled ankles by running on even surfaces when possible. Know your route and know where the dogs live. Almost every runner has had a problem with a dog. Most areas have leash laws, but always carry your phone. Snap a photo of the dog at large, or off leash, and text it and the address to your local law enforcement. They will remind the owners and the dog problems should diminish.

What should you do when you are forced to take time off due to an injury?

Try this:

Apply first aid for runners, or RICE.

Rest. Take time off from running. You can cross train to stay in condition if the activity does not aggravate the injured area.

Ice. Cold packs will reduce inflammation and swelling, especially when applied during the first 24 – 48 hours after onset.

Compression: Ace bandages, athletic tape, and compression socks will also help to support the affected area and reduce swelling.

Elevation: Put your feet up! The benefit is twofold. Elevation helps reduce swelling. In a runner's case, this is usually the feet and legs. You can't run if your feet are elevated, so this step also promotes rest.

If you don't see an improvement quickly, visit a health care professional to determine if you have a serious injury, and then follow their advice.

A quick guide to know when to take time off:

Take time off if weather conditions indicate injury is likely. Stay safe!

Take time off if you have an injury that is aggravated by working out. Sore muscles are not an injury. Learn to identify the difference.

Take time off if your training plan calls for a Rest Day. Don't assume you know more than the seasoned runners and coaches that have collaborated to develop training plans. If it says rest, then you should rest or cross train!

Take time off if your running shoes are worn out. Are your feet hurting? Did you examine your soles? Avoid an injury by taking time off until you have purchased new running shoes.

Take time off if you are dead. A head cold is not akin to death. You can, if you choose, continue to run while fighting a cold or sinus infection. In fact, running will keep everything else running! You may want to take along a handkerchief. Fold it in a cravat and tie it around your wrist to keep it handy.

Be wise. If the conditions outside are too hot or too slick and icy, don't run. You can use a treadmill if you have one, but don't risk injury.

No matter how difficult it may be to take time off, the rest may actually speed your recuperation and get you back out on the road running again.

Begin Again and Again

This trouble shooting tip is about starting over. It happens to all of us. We get injured or become ill. We have a change in life circumstances. We train hard for a race and then have trouble getting back into the swing of things once we have recovered from the race itself. Whatever the reason, everyone has times when they fall off the fitness wagon. Don't be discouraged – you have a chance to start over! There is no time like the present to begin training again.

Opportunities to begin training abound throughout the year. Perhaps, in spite of your best intentions, you failed to run through the late winter months. It's easy to become sidetracked during the holidays and cold weather. What better opportunity than the new year to begin again?

Make a New Year's Resolution to do better than last year. Be as specific or vague as you like, but determine to run more, smarter, or faster than you did the previous year.

Race season begins in the late spring. If you begin in January, you have plenty of time to get in condition for a spring 5K, 10K, or Half Marathon.

With spring on its way, it may feel okay to snuggle in warm layers of loose clothing, but that won't be the case when the temperatures start to climb. Look down the road a few weeks and plan to be get in shape by running now.

Not every runner takes time off in the winter. Summer can be so full of family vacations and activities that you might find yourself heading into fall a little sluggish and out of running condition. Determine to use running to offset those added calories that are inevitable in the later part of the year.

You began running before and you can begin running again. Transform your thinking. Don't tell yourself, "Oh, no! I quit running!" Rather, remind yourself that you are in it for the long haul. This is a lifetime sport. It's part of your lifestyle now. So, you had a little off season. Snow skiers and water skiers do, too. Yours just isn't as regularly scheduled as the skiers' seasons.

Don't panic. It will take time, but you'll get back in running shape. It will probably happen faster thank you expect.

You are not alone. I've had to start over more than a couple times. I am always surprised how quickly I settle in. The mileage adds up and soon I have forgotten that I ever took time off.

Try this:

Set a goal and make it known. Share your resolve with a friend who will help to hold you accountable, especially if that friend happens to be one of your running buddies.

If you have not yet participated in a race or fun run, now is a good time to register. It's that simple. The financial commitment and the fact that your name is on a list somewhere as a participant will encourage you to get moving. You may receive email updates and other social media encouragements from the race directors. This will build excitement as you anticipate race day and strive to be prepared to do your best.

Inventory your closet. Try on a few of those favorite warm weather items you haven't worn for a while. Perhaps that will be motivation enough. Squeeze into your swimsuit. It won't lie!

Start a group text with other runners to support and encourage one another by scheduling group runs or simply sharing your good and not so good running experiences.

Review your monthly mileage goal. Do you need to set a new goal? Write it down and begin filling in those blank spaces in your mileage log.

Your miles will start to add up before you know it!

My Feet Still Hurt

It's probably time for new shoes. Stop procrastinating and go shopping!

End of subject.

Section IV

Runners' Speech

Runners have a vocabulary all their own. As mentioned earlier in this book, we aren't the most patient of life's participants. We have a need for speed. Hence, the neglected cool downs and stretching, the constant comparing and obsession with pace and race results, and an abbreviated way of communicating.

The following pages contain a list of vocabulary terms often used by runners. Some will be familiar and others may surprise you. Some are comical while others are quite technical. All these terms have a purpose. A quick read through them will give you a glimpse into the life and mind of a runner. As you evolve as a runner, so will your speech. This list will help.

Enjoy!

The Runner's Vocabulary

Bonk – Hitting a virtual wall or running out of carbs and fluids during a race. It feels like a car running out of gas.

Carb Loading or Carbo Loading – A runner's excuse to eat a lot of pasta. In theory, it helps the runner prepare for a race by fueling and hydrating early. Truthfully? We just like carbohydrates.

Chafed – Yeah, it happens and we talk about it.

Cotton Mouth – What it feels like when you forgot your stick of gum.

Fartlek – Not what it sounds like. Similar to speed work. Alternating sprinting and recovery for short distances over a long run.

Fun Run – A race, usually 5K or 3.1 miles. It's not an oxymoron. It really is fun and you can walk if you must. It's a great place to get a PR.

Full – A marathon.

Half – Half marathon or 13.1 miles.

Hammies – Hamstring muscles.

Hill Work – Just like it sounds. Run uphill and jog down. Repeat. Repeat. Repeat.

Hydration – Drinking lots of fluids to avoid muscle cramps.

Long Run – This is the longest run of the week. The long run is typically performed at a slower pace than the other runs that week. It could be four miles or 24 miles, depending on the race distance. It's all relative.

Marathon – 26.2 miles.

Nemesis – Wind. Hills. Sleet. Stress injuries. Russian Olive trees in bloom.

Pace – The time it takes you to cover a specified distance. Usually a mile.

PB – Personal Best. Substitute term for PR.

PR – Personal Record. This can apply to pace, distance, or any other stat that the runner deems important.

RICE – Rest. Ice. Compression. Elevation.

Runners – Other runners. Track athletes. Very cool people. And our running shoes.

Short Run – Like the longest run of the week, only shortest … and faster.

Snot Rocket – aka Farmer Blow. The art of removing mucus from one's nostrils when no tissue paper or handkerchief is available.

Speed Work – A very short run, only faster, over and over with slower breaks in between.

Split – The pace at which you run smaller distances during a race or workout, ie., "My first half mile split was 5 minutes, but my second split was 4 minutes." (I wish!)

Tilt-a-Pottie – An outdoor portable toilet situated precariously on a road bank. It might tip over, but we don't care. It will have to do!

Vitamin I – Ibuprofen.

Conclusion

Congratulations! You are becoming a runner. Your experience as a runner will be unique to you. It will also be rewarding.

You will find that the running community, and it is quite large, is one of the most accepting and encouraging groups you will ever encounter. Perhaps it is because runners feel that they are misunderstood by non-runners or that they are excited to find a new friend who could possibly become a running buddy. Runners know how hard you are trying, because they were once beginners themselves. And let's face it, misery truly does love company. Runners don't care if you are slow or old. They aren't interested in your annual income. They are more curious about your running shoes than your sports car or vacation home – unless the vacation home would be a great place from which to go for a run and your sports car is a large SUV that could double as a relay race van.

Your doctor will be impressed with your improved blood pressure reading and lowered blood sugar levels.

Your family may join you or think you are crazy, but they will appreciate your efforts to be healthy on their behalf. Just be certain to control your enthusiastic running chatter amongst the non-running family members. They may think you are trying to force them into taking up the sport when you are only sharing your PR's, favorite shoes, and play-by-play long run experience. They aren't that interested.

Your heart will thank you by becoming stronger.

Your lungs will thank you when next you engage in another recreational activity. They won't let you down.

Your legs will thank you for their added strength, even though they may curse you when you've pushed them to their limits.

Your brain will be clearer. That's just how exercise works.

Your gift list and contents of your closet will evolve to include running apparel, gadgets, and shoes. Oh, the joy of new running shoes!

And … one day you will be pleasantly surprised when you meet someone new and as you shake hands you say, "I am a runner."

You are a runner!

About the Author

Carol M Green encourages women, especially grandmothers, to gain greater fitness by providing tips and inspiration to insure long years of joyful grand-parenting. She blogs as Running Granny Green. She explains ...

I began running at the tender age of 47, just prior to becoming a grandmother. I have always been involved in fitness programs of some kind or another, but running changed a lot of things.

Running broadened my horizons. I gained friends whom I would not have come to know without running. I refer to them as my running buddies. I began participating in fitness challenges and endurance activities from 5K's to sprint triathlons and half marathons. My favorite endurance challenge is a relay race where I share 180 miles of exhausting smelly misery with 11 of my running buddies.

Running improved my health. My blood pressure reading lowered. My endurance improved making other physical activities more enjoyable. My knees and ankles became stronger. (Yes, they did!)

Running improved my writing. I share things I have learned in effort to teach others. I have discovered so much value in running that I want to encourage others to lace up and run.

I am a wife, mother, and grandmother. I want to be able to enjoy those relationships for many years to come. Running is helping me accomplish that goal.

Bibliography

What Will You Wear?

"Spandex." Wikipedia. Wikimedia Foundation, 30 Apr. 2017. Web. 09 May 2017.

Follow a Plan

http://www.coolrunning.com/engine/2/2_3/181.shtml   Accessed May 2017.

http://www.mapmyrun.com/ Accessed May 2017.

https://runkeeper.com/ Accessed May 2017.

Read Something Inspirational

"Pinterest • The World's Catalog of Ideas." Pinterest. N.p., n.d. Web. 09 May 2017.

Take Time Off

http://www.andorrapediatrics.com/ap_folders/hand-outs/knowledge/rice.htm Accessed May 2017.

The Runner's Vocabulary

"Fartlek." Wikipedia. Wikimedia Foundation, 17 Apr. 2017. Web. 09 May 2017.

www.ingramcontent.com/pod-product-compliance
Lightning Source LLC
Chambersburg PA
CBHW072202280526
45788CB00002B/835